Community Helpers at Work

BOOKWORMS

A Day with a Doctor

By Katie Kawa

Cavendish Square

New York

Published in 2021 by Cavendish Square Publishing, LLC
243 5th Avenue, Suite 136, New York, NY 10016

First Edition

Website: cavendishsq.com

Cataloging-in-Publication Data

Names: Kawa, Katie.
Title: A day with a doctor / Katie Kawa.
Description: First edition. | New York : Cavendish Square, 2021. | Series: Community helpers at work | Includes index.
Identifiers: ISBN 9781502658067 (pbk.) | ISBN 9781502658081 (library bound) | ISBN 9781502658074 (6 pack) | ISBN 9781502658098 (ebook)
Subjects: LCSH: Physicians–Juvenile literature. | Medicine–Juvenile literature.
Classification: LCC R690.K27 2021 | DDC 610.69'5–dc23

Editor: Katie Kawa
Copy Editor: Nathan Heidelberger
Designer: Andrea Davison-Bartolotta

The photographs in this book are used by permission and through the courtesy of: Cover, p. 21 (bottom right) Monkey Business Images/Shutterstock.com; p. 5 Yakobchuk Viacheslav/Shutterstock.com; p. 7 ESB Professional/Shutterstock.com; p. 9 Octa corp/Shutterstock.com; p. 11 Erickson Stock/Shutterstock.com; p. 13 didesign021/Shutterstock.com; p. 15 Kamil Macniak/Shutterstock.com; p. 17 Happy Together/Shutterstock.com; p. 19 Inside Creative House/Shutterstock.com; p. 21 (top left) VGstockstudio/Shutterstock.com; p. 21 (top right) Standret/Shutterstock.com; p. 21 (bottom left) Andrey_Popov/Shutterstock.com; p. 23 fizkes/Shutterstock.com.

CPSIA compliance information: Batch #CS20CSQ: For further information contact Cavendish Square Publishing LLC, New York, New York, at 1-877-980-4450.

Printed in the United States of America

CONTENTS

Doctors on the Job

Doctors help many people in their **community**. They help sick people. They help people who are hurt. Doctors help them feel better. They have an important job to do!

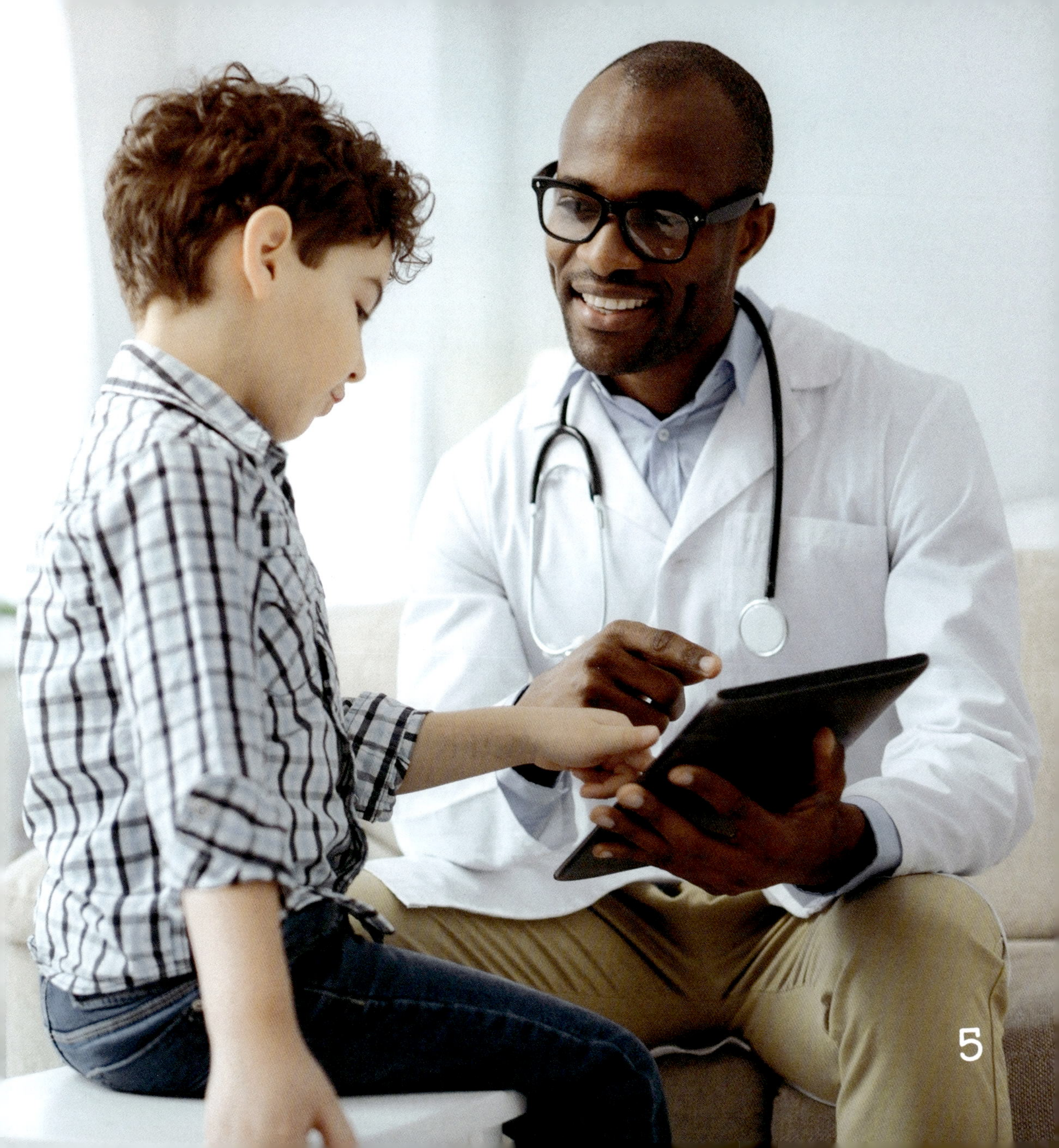

Doctors work in different places. A doctor might work in a hospital. This is a place people go when they're very sick or very badly hurt. Many doctors work in a hospital.

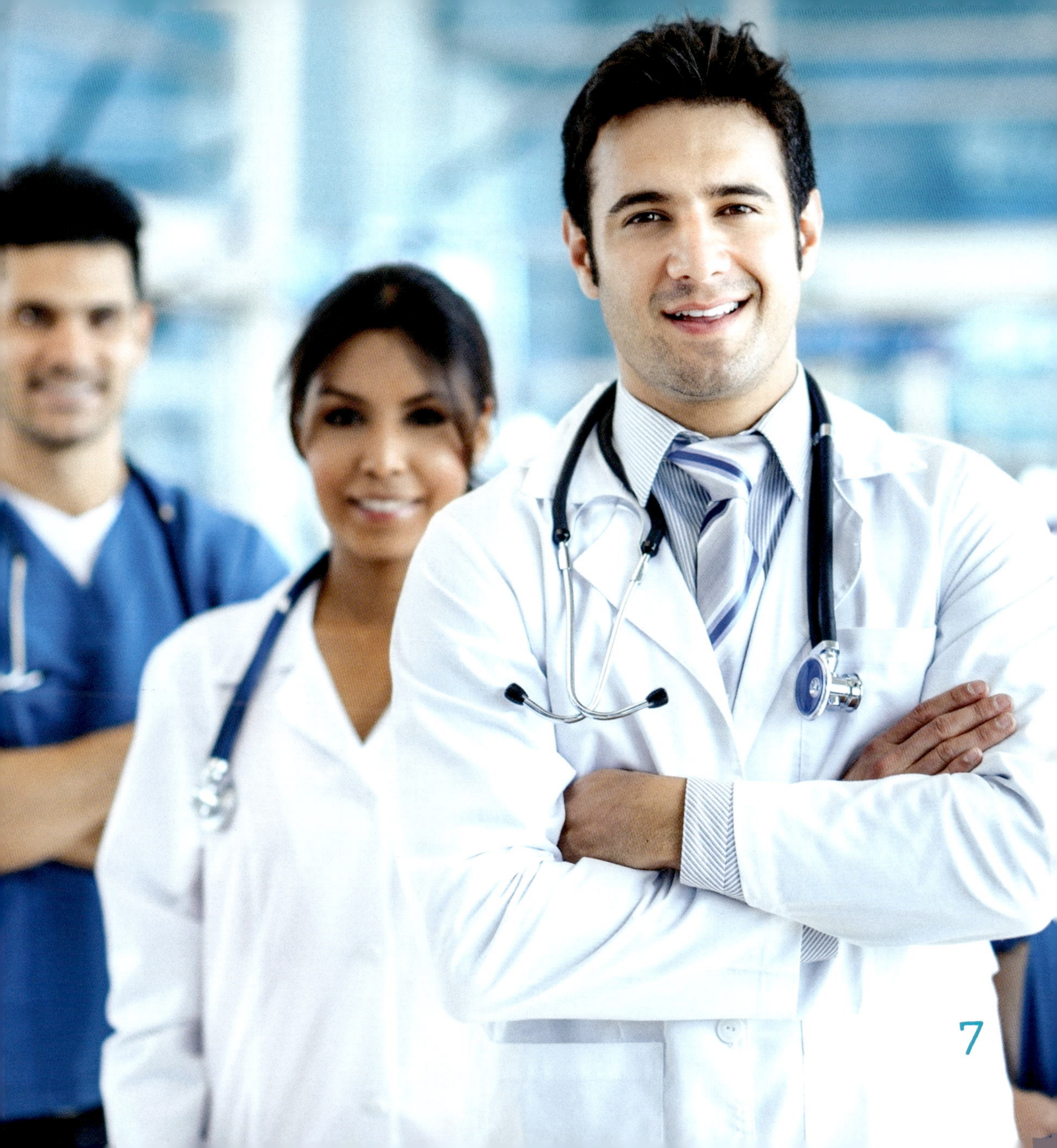

Some doctors have their own office. People visit the office when they're sick. Other doctors work in an office together. This is called a practice. The doctors help each other!

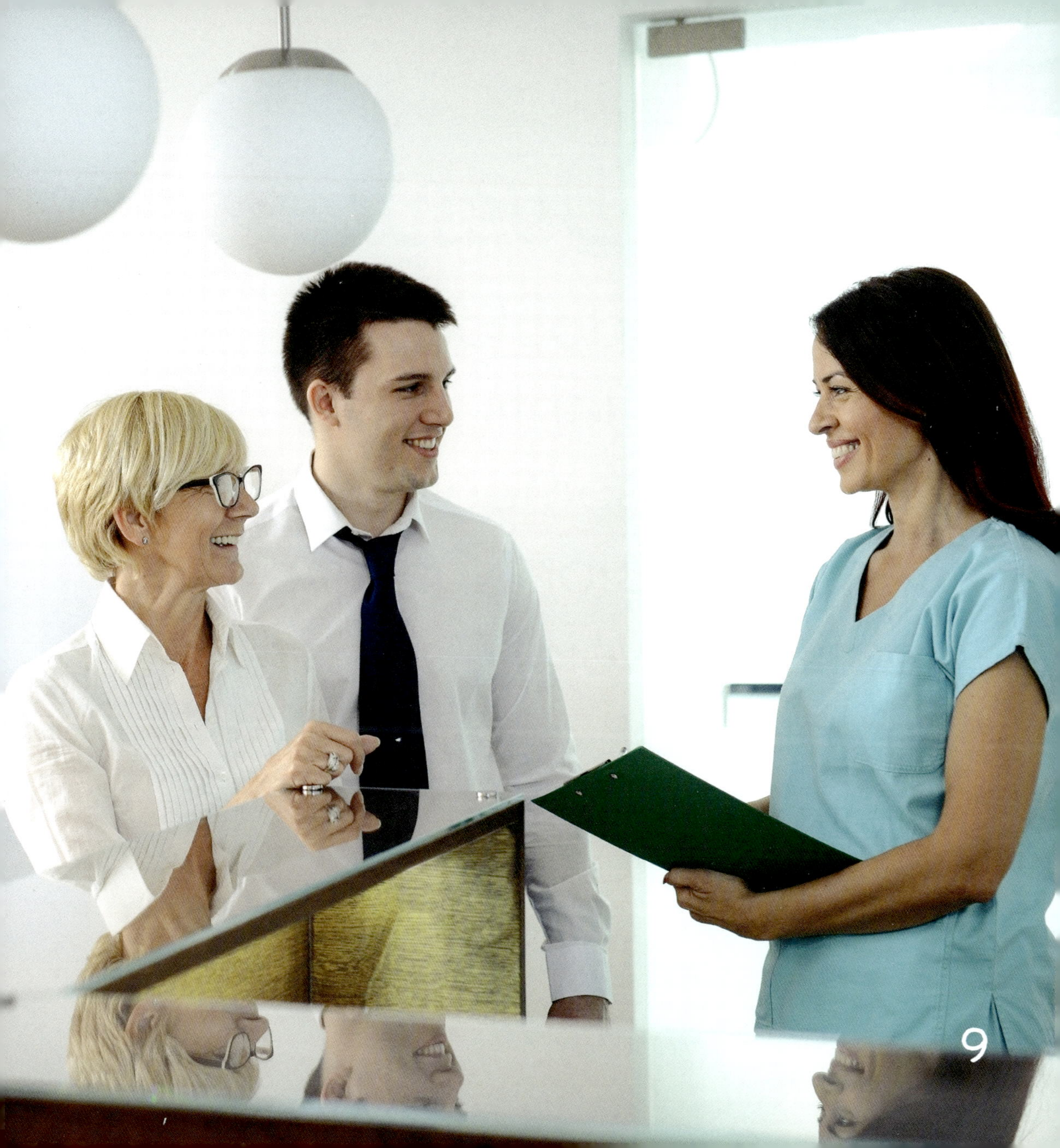

Seeing a Doctor

Nurses help doctors. They see patients first. A patient is someone who needs a doctor. Nurses check a patient's weight and **height**. They also ask questions about how the patient feels.

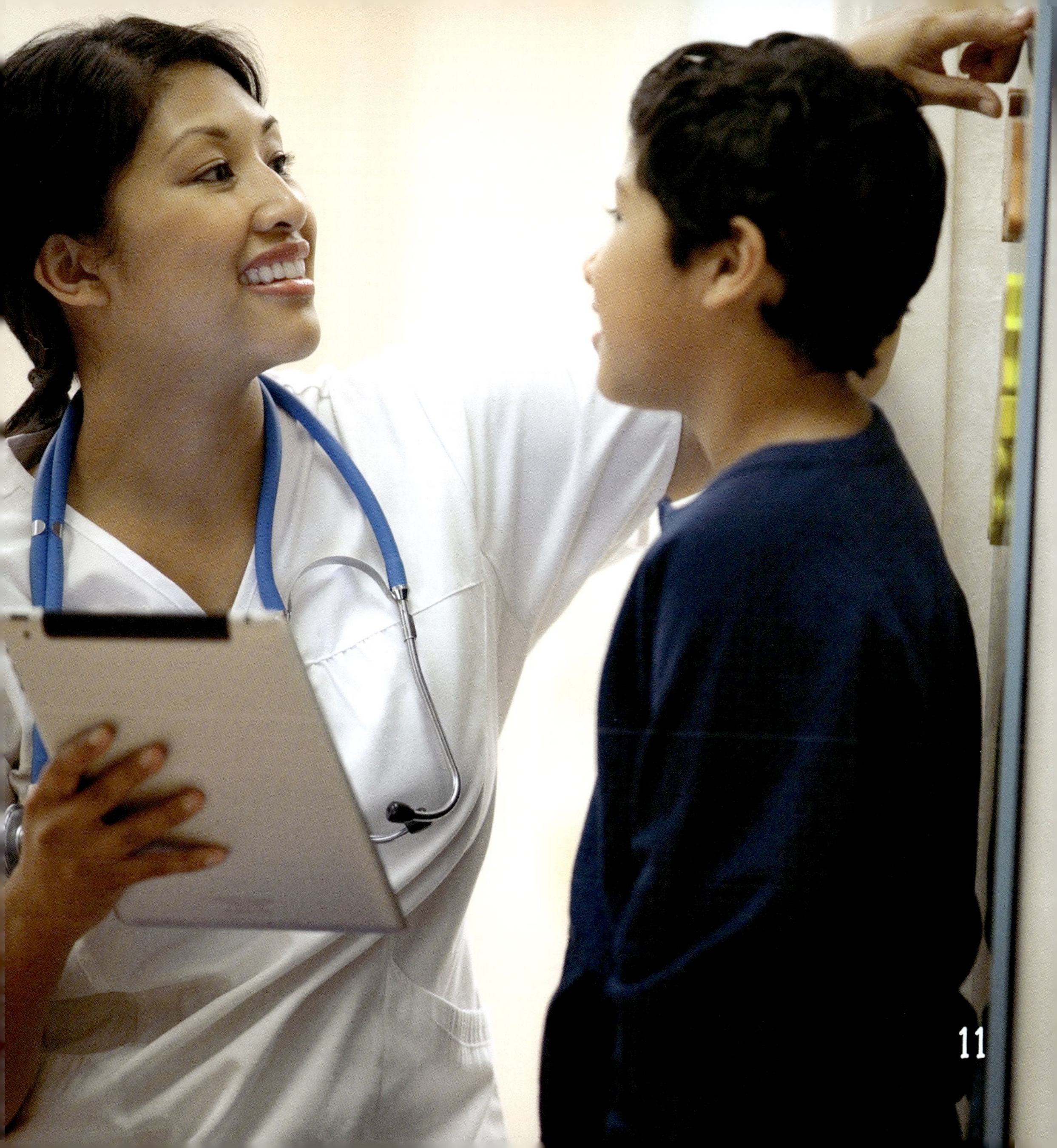

Then, a patient sees the doctor. They tell the doctor what's wrong. The doctor listens carefully. A doctor might listen to a patient's heart. They might also listen to a patient's breathing.

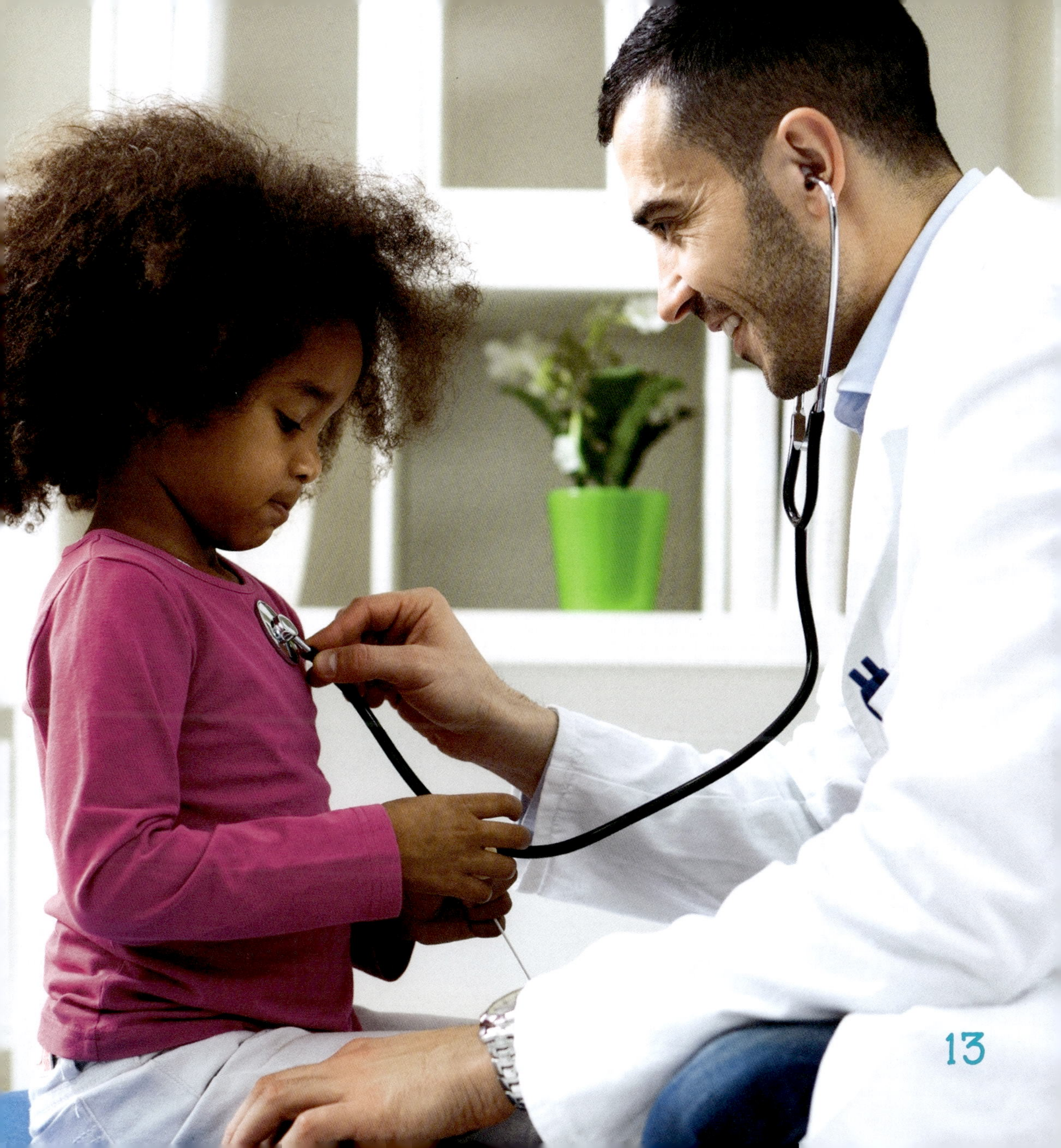

Doctors use different tools to find out what's wrong. They use a small light. They use this light to look into a person's ears, nose, and mouth. They use it to look at a person's eyes too.

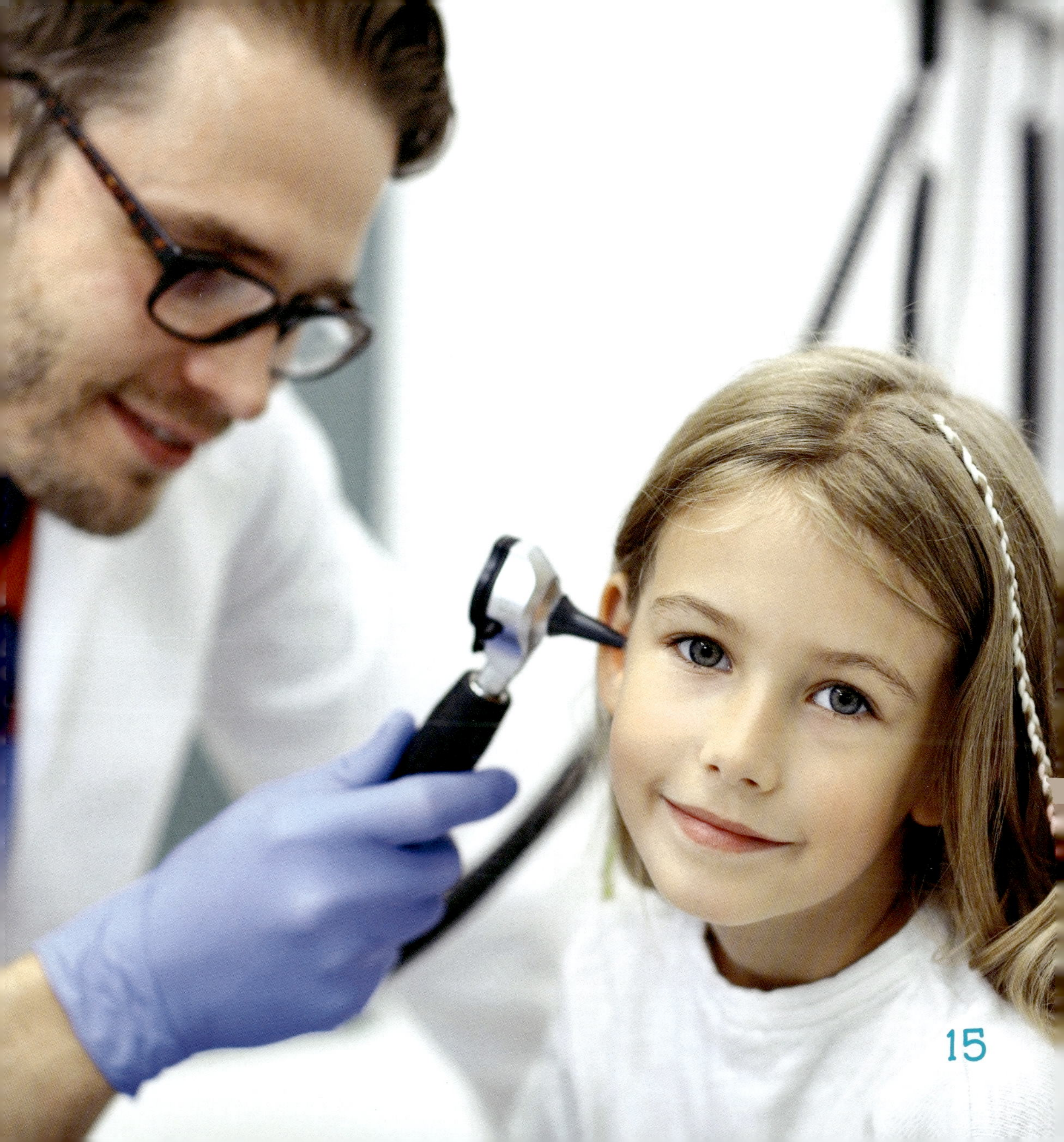

People see a doctor when they think they've broken a bone. A doctor uses X-rays to find out if a bone is broken. An X-ray is a picture that shows the inside of the body.

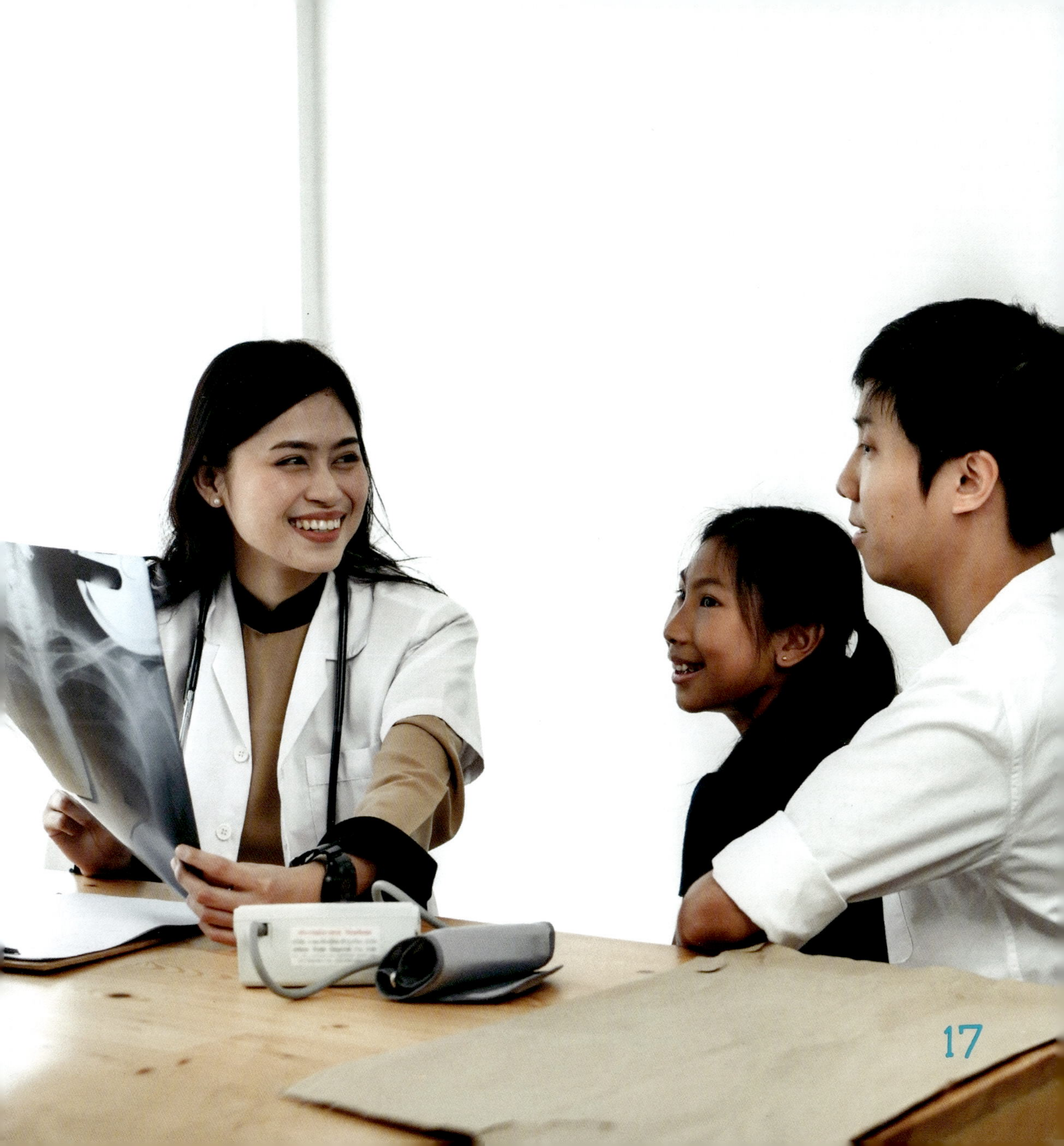

Doctors know how to help their patients. When someone is sick, a doctor can give them **medicine**. This can help them feel better. Doctors also give people shots. Shots keep people from getting sick.

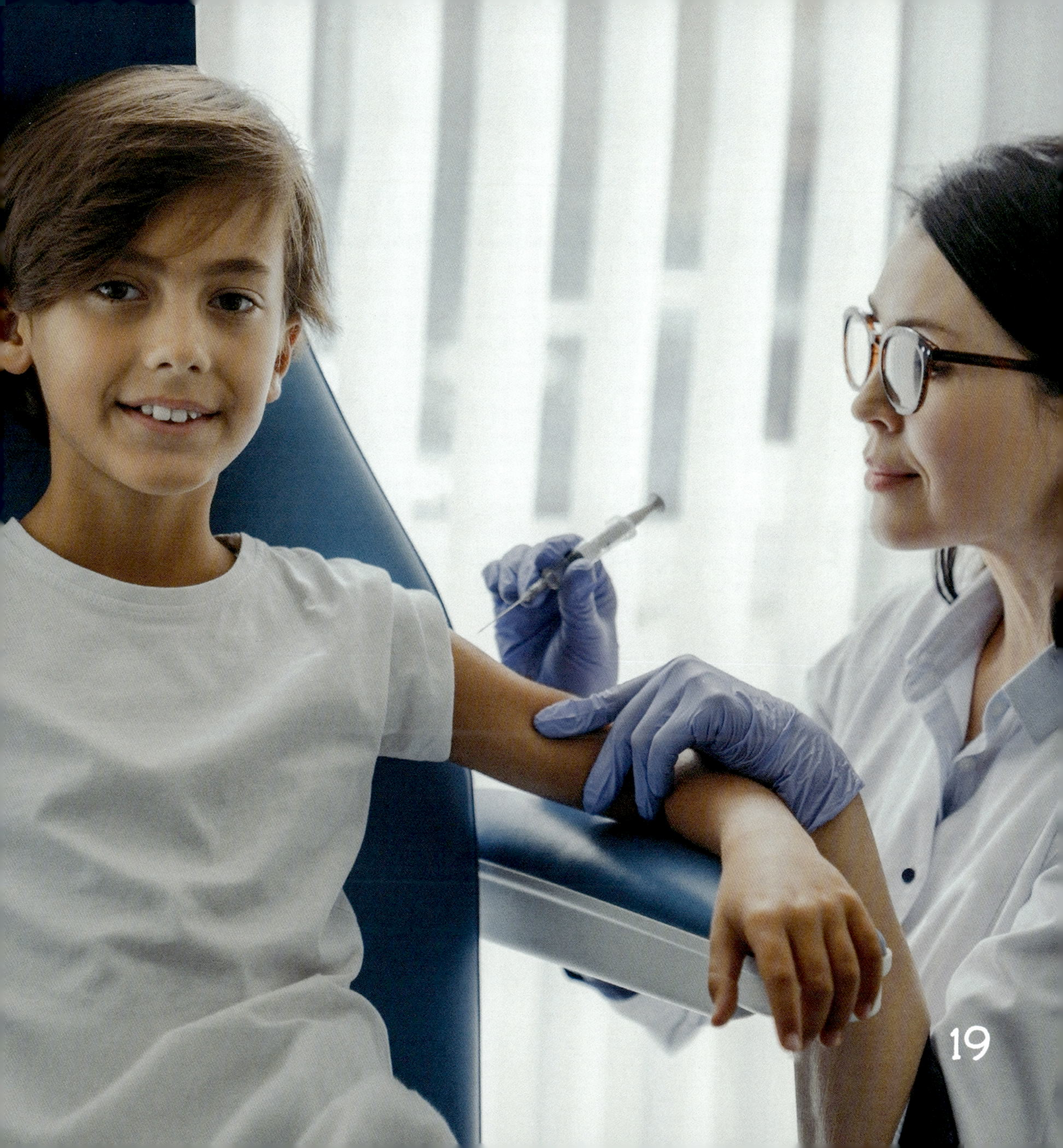

Different Kinds of Doctors

There are many different kinds of doctors! One kind of doctor looks at people's skin. Another kind of doctor looks at people's eyes. Some doctors only work with kids. Others only help older people.

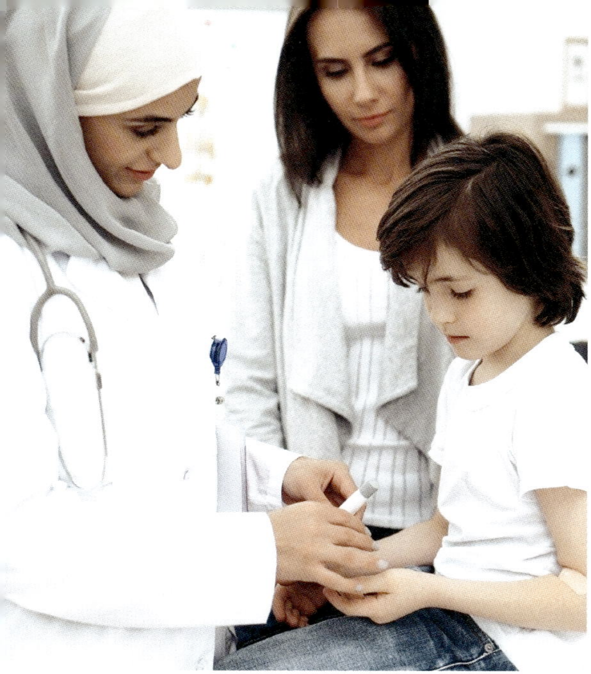
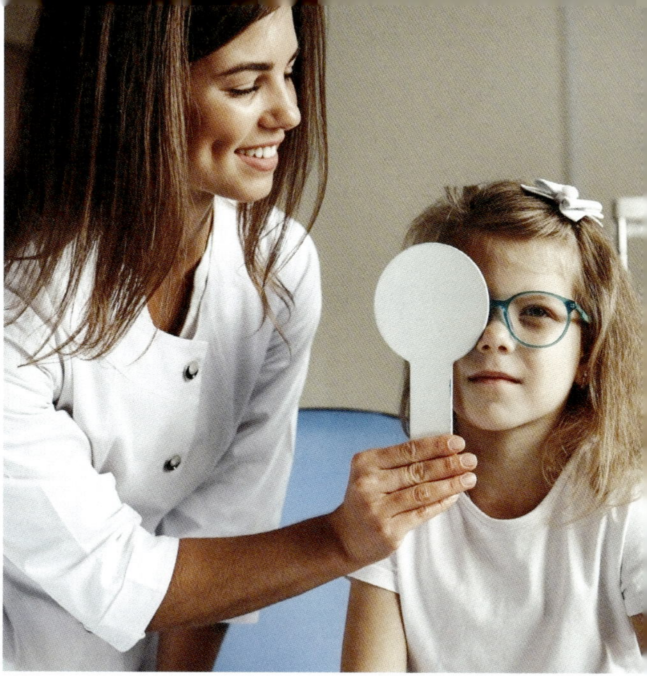
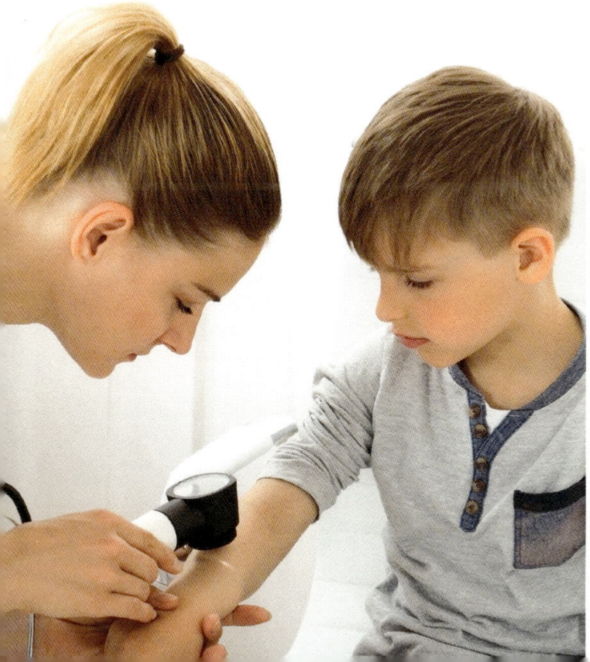
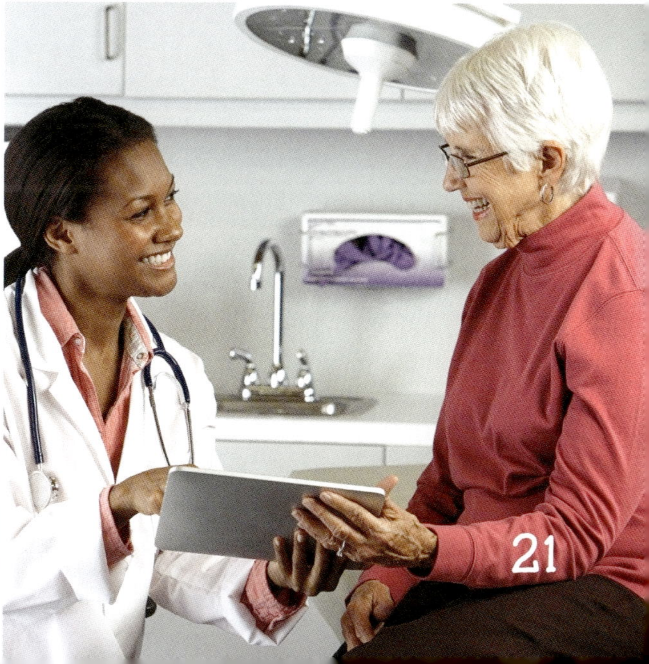

All kinds of doctors help people stay healthy and fit. They teach people how to take care of their body. They work hard to help people feel their best!

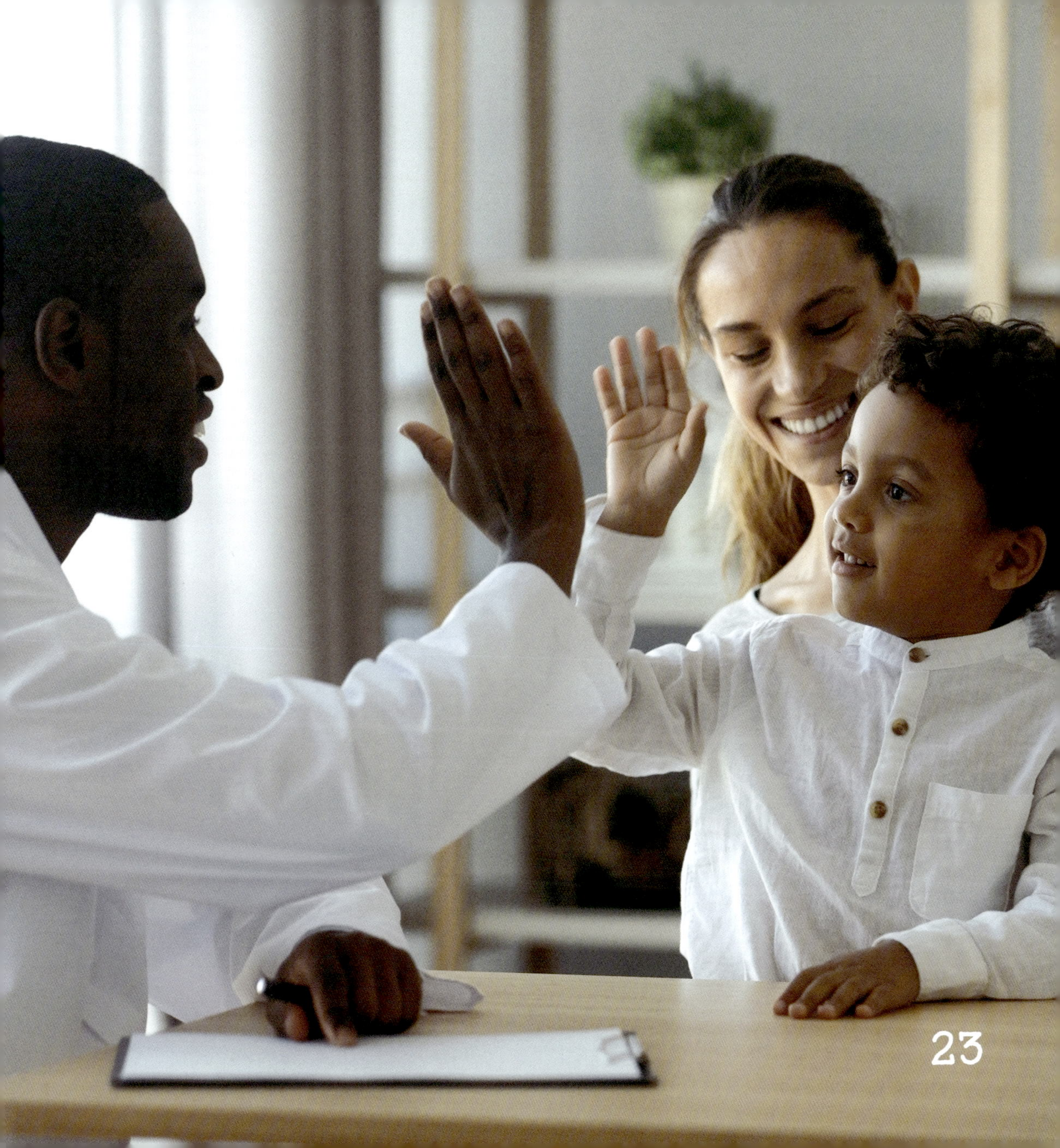

WORDS TO KNOW

community: An area where people live; a neighborhood.

height: How tall a person is.

medicine: Something a person takes to feel better when they are sick or hurting.

INDEX